Exploring The Mind-Gut-Immune Connection

Unraveling the Effects of Nutrition on our Brain, Microbiome, and Immune System

Dr. Stephanie C. McCarthy

Table of contents

Chapter 1. An Overview of the Mind-Gut-Immune Connection............ **6**

Recognizing the Mind-Gut-Immune Axis...........6

- Historical Context................................8

- Current Research Environment.................... 10

Chapter 2: The Gut Microbiome: An Invisible Orchestrator... **11**

The Brain-Gut Axis: A Two-Way Conversation...
11

The Gut-Immune Nexus and Stress...............12

Nutrition: Fueling a Healthy Relationship........ 12

Mindful Eating and Mindfulness...................... 13

Chapter 3. The Role of the Brain in Mental Health.. **14**

- The Emotional Neuroscience....................... 14

- The Effects of Stress on the Brain................ 16

Chapter 4. The Gut Microbiome: An Important Role in Overall Health................................ **18**

- What is the Gut Microbiome?.......................18

- Communication Between the Gut and the Brain...20

- Keeping a Healthy Microbiome.................... 22

Chapter 5. The Immune System: Protecting the Body from Infections................................ **25**

- Immune System Constituents...................... 25

How the immune system works...................... 27

The immune system and disease................... 28

- Immune Response to Pathogens.................. 29

- Immunomodulation and Autoimmunity..........32

Chapter 6. The Interplay Between the Mind, Gut, and Immune System..............................36

- Bidirectional Communication Pathways........36

Understanding and Harnessing Bidirectional Communication..40

- Psychoneuroimmunology: The Science of the Mind-Body Connection.....................................40

Chapter 7. How Diet and Lifestyle Influence Mental and Physical Health.......................45

- Effects of Exercise on the Mind and Body....45

How Much Physical Activity Is Enough?.........47

- Circadian Rhythms and Sleep......................48

Chapter 8: Healthy Mind, Gut, and Immune System Strategies.......................................50

- Stress Reduction Techniques.......................50

Systems of assistance....................................58

Strategies to obtain Stress Management........58

Adults are also affected by ADHD...................60

ADHD Symptoms...62

What Are the Causes of ADHD?.....................63

ADHD Diagnosis in Adults.............................63

ADHD Complications in Adults.......................64

Treatments for ADHD.....................................64

Chapter 9: The Beneficial Effects of Probiotics on Mental Health...................................66

- Knowledge of Probiotics and Prebiotics.......66

Mood Disorders and Probiotics......................69

- Clinical Use of Probiotics............................70

Chapter 10: The Role of Antioxidants in Promoting Mental and Gut Health..................72

- Inflammation and Oxidative Stress...............72

- Food Antioxidants.. 74

- Supplementation with antioxidants.............. 76

Chapter 11. Stress Reduction Techniques for a Healthy Mind and Body....................................... 78

Cognitive Behavioral Therapy (CBT).............. 78

- Neurofeedback and biofeedback.................. 80

Chapter 12: Sleep Hygiene: Making Rest a Priority for a Healthy Mind and Immune System. 82

- The Sleep Science...82

Chapter 13: Hydration and Its Effects on Mental and Physical Health... 84

- Water and Cognitive Function.......................84

- Electrolyte Stability..85

Chapter 14: Adopting a Balanced Diet for a Strong Mind, Gut, and Immune System........... 87

- The Mediterranean Diet................................ 87

- Plant-Based Diets... 91

- Personalized Nutrition...................................96

Chapter 15: The Role of Exercise in Promoting Mental and Physical Well-being....................... 99

- Types of Exercise and Their Benefits........... 99

- Exercise and Neuroplasticity......................101

- Exercise Prescription.................................. 103

Conclusion... 105

Chapter 1. An Overview of the Mind-Gut-Immune Connection

Recognizing the Mind-Gut-Immune Axis

The mind-gut-immune axis is a network of bidirectional communication that connects the central nervous system, the enteric nervous system, and the immune system. This network includes not only anatomical communication channels, but also endocrine, humoral, metabolic, and immunological communication routes. The gut-brain axis is a bidirectional communication network that connects the enteric and central nervous systems and is a critical component of the mind-gut-immune axis. The brain may regulate intestinal processes, including the activation of functional immunity effector cells, and the gut can influence mood, cognition, and mental health.

The gut microbiome is important in the mind-gut-immune axis because it regulates both the gut-brain axis and the immune system. The gut microbiota may communicate with the brain via neuronal, endocrine, immunological, and humoral pathways, and it can also impact the immune system via metabolites and other signaling molecules. Through the creation of neurotransmitters and other signaling molecules that may penetrate the blood-brain barrier, the gut microbiota can also impact mood, cognition, and mental health.

The immune system is an essential component of the mind-gut-immune axis because it protects the body from illnesses and maintains general health. Through numerous signaling molecules, the immune system may interact with the brain and the stomach, and it can also be impacted by the gut microbiota[3].

Understanding the mind-gut-immune axis is critical for general health and illness prevention. Individuals may promote a healthy mind, stomach, and immune system and lower their chance of acquiring numerous mental and physical health disorders by adopting smart food and lifestyle choices.

- Historical Context

The mind-gut immune link has been studied since at least the seventeenth century, with researchers and medical professionals investigating the connections between the gut, mind, and emotions. Here are some major breakthroughs in our understanding of the mind-gut immunological connection:

1. Eighteenth and nineteenth centuries: The focus was on the link between the stomach and emotions during this time period. Doctors and patients both believed in the deep links between the stomach and the mind, and they tried a variety of techniques to learn more about these interactions. Their understanding was restricted, however, by a lack of microbiological and psychological approaches to comprehending body interactions.

2. Twentieth century: In the early twentieth century, researchers began to investigate the relationship between the stomach and the mind. They not only connected gut activity to emotions, but they also predicted possible societal advantages if the general population maintained excellent gut health. Memoirs from this time period described a complicated relationship between the mind, stomach, and emotions.

3. Mid-twentieth century: The gut-brain axis notion gained hold, with researchers focused on connection between the digestive organs and the brain. At times, the emphasis was on the connectivity of the gut and mind, but at other times, researchers isolated and concentrated on specific parts of the stomach. The pendulum continued to swing back and forth, with studies relating gut behavior to emotions and investigating the possible societal advantages of good gut health.

4. Late twentieth and twenty-first centuries: Our understanding of the mind-gut immunological link has advanced dramatically in recent decades. With

the growth of microbiome research and the discovery of the human microbiome, we now have a better knowledge of the connections between the gut, mind, and immune system. The emphasis has switched from merely correlating gut activity to emotions to investigating the intricate communication networks that exist between the gut bacteria, the brain, and the immune system.

Researchers have utilized many techniques and methodologies to explore the connections between the gut, brain, and emotions throughout the history of the mind-gut immunological link. These techniques have included investigating historical and current perspectives on gut-mind-environment connections, as well as the consequences of these interactions for human health and well-being.

- Current Research Environment

The complex interplay between the mind, stomach, and immune system, known as the "mind-gut-immune connection," has arisen as a fascinating topic of scientific investigation. Researchers have delved into the interesting processes that explain this intricate interaction during the last decade, revealing a plethora of evidence highlighting the significant influence of mental and emotional well-being on gut health and immune function.

Chapter 2: The Gut Microbiome: An Invisible Orchestrator

The gut microbiome, a varied population of billions of bacteria living in the intestines, is at the center of the mind-gut-immune relationship. These microbial inhabitants play an important role in digestive health, nutrition absorption regulation, and immune response regulation. Dysbiosis, or disruptions in the gut microbiome, has been related to a variety of health issues, including inflammatory bowel disease, irritable bowel syndrome, and even autoimmune illnesses.

The Brain-Gut Axis: A Two-Way Conversation

The brain and gut are continually talking with one another via the brain-gut axis, a bidirectional neuronal network. The brain may regulate gut

motility, digestion, and the makeup of the gut
microbiota thanks to this complicated
communication network. The stomach, on the other
hand, sends messages to the brain, which influences
emotions, stress perception, and even behavior.

The Gut-Immune Nexus and Stress

Stress, an ever-present factor in modern life, has been
identified as an important modulator of the
mind-gut-immune relationship. Chronic stress may
wreak havoc on the delicate balance of the gut
microbiota, resulting in increased intestinal
permeability and inflammation. This, in turn, can
result in excessive immune responses, which can
contribute to the development of a variety of health
issues such as allergies, asthma, and autoimmune
disorders.

Nutrition: Fueling a Healthy Relationship

The food we eat has a significant impact on the gut flora and the mind-gut-immune relationship. A diet abundant in processed foods, sugary drinks, and artificial sweeteners has been found to foster a diversified and healthy gut microbiome, but a diet high in fruits, vegetables, whole grains, and fermented foods can lead to dysbiosis.

Mindful Eating and Mindfulness

Mindfulness, defined as the practice of concentrating one's attention on the present moment without judgment, has emerged as a potent technique for strengthening the mind-gut-immune link. Mindful eating, or paying attention to the sensory signals of eating without interruptions, can aid in the regulation of eating habits, the reduction of stress-induced overeating, and the improvement of nutritional absorption.

Chapter 3. The Role of the Brain in Mental Health

- The Emotional Neuroscience

Emotional neuroscience is a complex and dynamic discipline that investigates the link between the brain, emotions, and the immune system. The immune response is also a vital component of the body's capacity to respond to stimuli and sustain general health. Emotions are described as "an essential part of the process of an organism's interaction with stimuli." The stomach is a crucial organ in the management of emotional behavior, according to research, and evidence is developing suggesting the immune system plays a substantial role in regulating emotional behavior.

The brain is the key organ in charge of emotion processing and controlling the body's reaction to emotional inputs. The limbic system, which comprises the amygdala, hippocampus, and hypothalamus, is an important brain area involved in emotional processing. The prefrontal cortex, which is in charge of higher-order cognitive tasks, is also important in controlling emotional reactions and behavior.

The immune system is a complex network of cells, tissues, and organs that work together to protect the body against outside invaders and to keep it healthy. The immune system and the brain are intertwined, according to research, and the immune system can impact emotional behavior. Immune cells, for example, can govern emotional behavior by modifying blood composition and the body's reaction to emotional stimuli.

The gut is also an important organ in the regulation of emotional behavior, and new data reveals that the gut microbiota is important in controlling emotional responses. The gut-brain axis is a bidirectional communication pathway that connects the gut and the brain, and studies have revealed that gut bacteria can influence emotional behavior by creating neurotransmitters and other signaling chemicals that affect the brain.

- The Effects of Stress on the Brain

Stress is a normal reaction to adversity, but persistent stress can have harmful consequences on the brain, such as poor memory, lower cognitive function, and an increased risk of mental illness. Because stress may alter the gut microbiota and immune system, the impact of stress on the brain is an important component of the mind-gut immunological relationship.

Chronic stress can cause an increase in cortisol production, a hormone that can impair brain function in a variety of ways. Cortisol can impair synapse control, resulting in a lack of sociability and avoidance of social contacts. Chronic stress can also cause the prefrontal cortex, the part of the brain responsible for memory and learning, to atrophy. Furthermore, stress can increase the size of the amygdala, making the brain more vulnerable to stress and creating a vicious cycle of fight-or-flight reactions.

The effects of stress on the brain can also have an impact on the gut microbiota and immune system. Chronic stress can alter the gut microbiota, resulting in a decrease in helpful bacteria and an increase in dangerous bacteria. These modifications can cause inflammation and immunological dysregulation, both of which can contribute to the development of chronic illnesses.

Mindfulness meditation, exercise, and relaxation practices, for example, can help alleviate the detrimental effects of stress on the brain, stomach, and immune system. Mindfulness-based eating and stress-reduction strategies can also help maintain a healthy gut flora and immune system.

Chapter 4. The Gut Microbiome: An Important Role in Overall Health

- What is the Gut Microbiome?

The gut microbiome, also known as the gut microbiota or gut flora, is a varied community of microorganisms that live in the digestive tracts of animals, including humans[1][3]. It includes bacteria, archaea, fungus, and viruses. This complex ecosystem, which mostly inhabits the gastrointestinal (GI) tract, is important in a variety of physiological activities and has a significant influence on human health.

Diversity and composition

The gut microbiota is extraordinarily varied, with the colon having the greatest microbial density of any human-associated microbial community examined thus far, with between 300 and 1000 distinct species[1]. While bacteria are the most abundant and well-studied component, the gut microbiota also includes archaea, fungi, viruses, and other species. The microbial makeup of the digestive system varies by area, with the colon having the highest microbial density.

Features

The gut microbiota performs a variety of critical activities, including:

- Metabolism: The microbiota is necessary for metabolizing dietary and medicinal substances, harvesting energy from food, and generating critical vitamins and nutrients.
- Immune Function: It is involved in immune system development and regulation, assisting in immunological homeostasis and protecting against pathogens.
- Gut-Brain Axis: The gut microbiota regulates brain function and behavior via the gut-brain axis, with new research emphasizing its involvement in mood, cognition, and mental health.

- Intestinal Barrier Function: It promotes gut health and integrity by contributing to the preservation of the intestinal epithelium and the strengthening of biochemical barriers inside the gut.

Clinical Consequences

The gut microbiome has been linked to a variety of health problems, and its dysregulation has been linked to illnesses such as gastrointestinal disorders, metabolic disorders, and immune-related ailments. Dysbiosis, or dysbiosis of the normal gut microbiota, has been associated to illnesses such as inflammatory bowel disease (IBD), irritable bowel syndrome (IBS), obesity, type 2 diabetes, and atopy.

- Communication Between the Gut and the Brain

The gut-brain axis is a bidirectional communication network that connects the enteric and central nervous systems and allows information to be exchanged between the gut and the brain. This network is not just anatomical, but it also includes endocrine, humoral, metabolic, and immunological communication pathways. The stomach and brain are physically and biochemically linked in a variety of ways, and they may impact each other's health.

Physical and Biochemical Relationships

- Vagus Nerve and Nervous System: The vagus nerve, one of the largest nerves linking the stomach and brain, plays an important role in signal transmission in both directions. It allows bidirectional communication by sending afferent signals from the stomach to the brain and efferent signals from the brain to the gut.

- Neurotransmitter-Receptor Sites: Neurologically active chemicals generated by the gut microbiota can influence brain function by modulating neurotransmitter synthesis, metabolism, and transmission. Microbes in the stomach, for example, convert the amino acid tryptophan into serotonin and other metabolites, hence controlling serotonin levels in the brain.

- Hormonal and Immune Pathways: The gut-brain axis also includes the autonomic nervous system, the hypothalamic-pituitary-adrenal (HPA) axis, and nerves within the gastrointestinal tract, all of which connect the gut and the brain, allowing intestinal activities, immune function, and mood regulation to be influenced.

Impact on Health

The gut-brain axis has been linked to a variety of health-related issues, including emotion, cognition, mental health, and gastrointestinal function. Clinical, epidemiological, and immunological data shows that the enteric microbiota has a large and profound impact on the gut-brain interaction, altering mental state, affective control, neuromuscular function, and HPA axis regulation.

Nutrition's Role

Nutrition is crucial in maintaining the health of the gut-brain axis. Certain nutrients, such as omega-3 fats, fermented foods, and high-fiber diets, have been found to boost beneficial bacteria in the stomach and promote brain health[1]. These foods can help maintain a healthy gut flora, which in turn helps the gut-brain axis communicate and operate.

- Keeping a Healthy Microbiome

Maintaining a healthy gut microbiome is critical for general health since the gut microbiota is involved in a variety of physiological activities such as metabolism, immunological function, and even mental health. According to the sources, the following are some critical techniques for keeping a healthy microbiome:

1. Dietary Fiber and Polyphenols: A diet high in fiber and plant polyphenols can help maintain a healthy gut microbiota. These components may be found in fruits, vegetables, whole grains, and legumes, and they provide nourishment for good gut bacteria.

2. Probiotics and Fermented Foods: Probiotics, which are live beneficial bacteria, can aid in the colonization of the gut with helpful germs. Fermented foods, such as yogurt, kefir, and kimchi, are high in probiotics and can help to maintain a varied microbiome.

3. **Avoid Processed Foods and Excess Sugar:** Processed foods and those high in refined sugars can have a deleterious influence on the gut microbiota, encouraging the growth of dangerous bacteria. Limiting your intake of certain items can help you keep your microbiome healthy.

4. **Regular Physical exercise:** Physical exercise has been linked to a more diversified and healthier gut microbiota. Incorporating frequent exercise into your regimen can help the microbiota's general health.

5. **Stress Management and Sleep:** Chronic stress and lack of sleep might affect the gut microbiome's homeostasis. Stress-relieving activities and emphasizing quality sleep can have a good influence on the microbiota.

6. **Avoiding Unnecessary Antibiotics:** Antibiotics have a major influence on the gut microbiome, frequently resulting in a temporary decrease of microbial diversity. To prevent altering the microbiota, antibiotics should be used sparingly and only when absolutely necessary[3].

By implementing these tactics into your daily routine, you may improve the health and variety of your gut microbiome, which can contribute to your general well-being and health.

Chapter 5. The Immune System: Protecting the Body from Infections

- Immune System Constituents

The immune system is a complex network of cells, tissues, and organs that collaborate to protect the body against infection and illness. It is a highly specialized system capable of recognizing and eliminating a wide spectrum of invaders such as bacteria, viruses, fungus, and parasites.

The basic components of the immune system are as follows:

- White blood cells (WBCs): WBCs are the immune system's major cells. They are produced in the bone marrow and circulate through the blood and lymphatic system. WBCs are classified into five categories, each with a distinct function:

- Neutrophils: The most prevalent form of WBC is neutrophils. They are phagocytes, which engulf and kill foreign intruders.

- Lymphocytes: Lymphocytes are in charge of particular immunity, meaning they can recall and kill specific intruders. Lymphocytes are classified into two types: B cells and T cells.

- B cells: B cells are responsible for the production of antibodies, which are proteins that attach to foreign invaders and mark them for destruction.

- T cells: T cells destroy contaminated cells and aid in immune response regulation.

- Monocytes: Another kind of phagocyte is the monocyte. When they infiltrate tissues, they mature into macrophages.

- Macrophages: Macrophages are phagocytes that engulf and kill invading organisms. They also aid in the removal of dead cells and debris.

- Antibodies: Antibodies are B-cell proteins that bind to certain foreign invaders. This identifies the intruders for elimination by other immune system cells.

- **Complement system:** The complement system is a collection of proteins that aid in the destruction of foreign invaders. It also aids in the activation of other immune system cells.
- **Lymph nodes:** Lymph nodes are little bean-shaped structures found all over the body. They filter the lymph, a transparent fluid containing white blood cells. Lymph nodes aid in the capture and destruction of foreign invaders.
- **Thymus:** The thymus is a small organ in the chest. It is in charge of T cell maturation.
- **Spleen:** The spleen is an organ in the upper left quadrant of the belly. It filters the blood and aids in the destruction of foreign invaders.

How the immune system works

The immune system is constantly working to protect the body from infection. When a foreign invader enters the body, the immune system goes through a series of steps to destroy it. These steps include:

1. Recognition: The immune system must first recognize the foreign invader as being foreign. This is done by special proteins on the surfaces of cells called antigen-presenting cells (APCs).

2. Activation: Once the foreign invader is recognized, the immune system is activated. This involves the activation of B cells and T cells.

3. Effector response: The activated B cells and T cells produce antibodies and other immune factors that destroy the foreign invader.

4. Memory formation: The immune system also remembers the foreign invader so that it can quickly attack it again if it enters the body again. This is called memory immunity.

The immune system and disease

The immune system is very effective at protecting the body from infection, but sometimes it makes mistakes. These mistakes can lead to autoimmune diseases, in which the immune system attacks the body's own tissues. The immune system can also be weakened by certain diseases, such as cancer and AIDS.

- Immune Response to Pathogens

The immune system is a complex and multifaceted defense mechanism that protects the body from a wide range of pathogens, including bacteria, viruses, fungi, and parasites. When a pathogen enters the body, it triggers a cascade of events known as the immune response, which aims to eliminate the invader and restore homeostasis.

The specific type of immune response elicited depends on the nature of the pathogen. Here's a breakdown of the immune response to different types of pathogens:

Pathogen	Immune Response
Bacteria	Neutrophils, macrophages, antibodies
Viruses	T cells, interferon, antibodies
Fungi	Neutrophils, macrophages, antibodies
Parasites	Eosinophils, antibodies

Bacteria

Bacteria are single-celled prokaryotic organisms that can cause a variety of infections, ranging from mild to life-threatening. The immune system's primary defense against bacteria involves neutrophils, which are phagocytic cells that engulf and destroy the invaders. Macrophages, another type of phagocyte, also play a crucial role in bacterial elimination. Additionally, antibodies produced by B lymphocytes bind to the bacteria, marking them for destruction by other immune cells.

Viruses

Viruses are much smaller and simpler than bacteria, lacking their own cellular machinery. They invade host cells and hijack their machinery to replicate and spread. The immune response to viruses primarily involves T cells, which can recognize and kill infected cells. Interferon, a signaling molecule produced by infected cells, helps to prevent the spread of the virus to neighboring cells. Antibodies also play a role in viral immunity by neutralizing the virus particles, preventing them from infecting new cells.

Fungi

Fungal infections can range from superficial skin infections to invasive systemic infections. The immune response to fungi involves neutrophils and macrophages, similar to the response against bacteria. Antibodies also contribute to fungal clearance by opsonizing the fungi, making them more susceptible to phagocytosis.

Parasites

Parasites are multicellular organisms that live and feed off other organisms. The immune response to parasites is often characterized by eosinophilia, an increase in the number of eosinophils, a type of white blood cell specialized in combating parasitic infections. Antibodies also play a role in parasite elimination by targeting the parasite's surface antigens.

The immune response to pathogens is a complex and dynamic process that involves a coordinated interplay of various immune cells and molecules. Understanding the mechanisms underlying the immune response is crucial for developing effective vaccines and treatments for infectious diseases.

-   Immunomodulation and Autoimmunity.

The immune system, our body's defense against pathogens and foreign substances, is a finely tuned mechanism that must maintain a delicate balance between protecting the body and avoiding self-destruction. Immunomodulation refers to the process of regulating the immune system's response, either boosting or suppressing it, to achieve a desired outcome.

Autoimmunity: When the Immune System Attacks Itself

Autoimmunity arises when the immune system mistakenly identifies the body's own healthy tissues as foreign invaders and launches an attack against them. This misguided attack leads to a range of autoimmune diseases, including rheumatoid arthritis, lupus, and multiple sclerosis.

Immunomodulation in Autoimmunity: Restoring Balance

In the context of autoimmunity, immunomodulation aims to restore the immune system's balance, preventing it from attacking healthy tissues. This can be achieved through various approaches, including:

1. **Suppressing the Overall Immune Response:** Medications such as corticosteroids and immunosuppressants can broadly suppress the immune system, reducing its overall activity and calming the autoimmune attack.

2. **Targeting Specific Immune Cells or Molecules:** Newer therapies, such as monoclonal antibodies, target specific immune cells or molecules involved in the autoimmune process, providing more precise control over the immune response.

3. **Promoting Tolerance to Self-Antigens:** Induction of tolerance to the self-antigens that the immune system is attacking is another promising approach, preventing the immune system from recognizing these antigens as foreign.

Challenges in Immunomodulation

Immunomodulation is a complex process, and striking the right balance is crucial. Excessive immunosuppression can leave the body vulnerable to infections, while insufficient suppression may not adequately control the autoimmune disease.

<u>Personalized Immunomodulation</u>

Individual variability in the immune system and the underlying autoimmune disease necessitates personalized immunomodulation strategies. Factors such as the specific autoimmune disease, the severity of symptoms, and the patient's overall health status must be considered when tailoring treatment plans.

<u>Immunomodulation: A Promising Path for Autoimmune Therapies</u>

Immunomodulation has revolutionized the treatment of autoimmune diseases, providing effective tools to manage these complex conditions. With ongoing research and advancements in personalized medicine, immunomodulation holds promise for further improving the lives of individuals with autoimmune diseases.

Chapter 6. The Interplay Between the Mind, Gut, and Immune System

- Bidirectional Communication Pathways.

Within the intricate tapestry of the human body, a symphony of communication is constantly flowing, connecting and coordinating diverse systems to maintain health and well-being. These communication pathways, bidirectional in nature, allow for the exchange of signals and information, ensuring that the body functions as a cohesive unit.

The Gut-Brain Axis: A Nerve-Gut Symphony

At the forefront of bidirectional communication stands the gut-brain axis, a direct neural highway connecting the enteric nervous system (ENS) within the gut to the central nervous system (CNS) in the brain. This intricate network of nerves, neurotransmitters, and hormones enables a constant dialogue between the gut and the brain, influencing emotions, behavior, and overall health.

Signals from the gut, such as those triggered by the gut microbiome, travel along the vagus nerve to the brain, influencing mood, stress perception, and even cognitive function. Conversely, the brain can exert control over the gut, modulating digestion, gut motility, and the permeability of the intestinal lining.

The Immune-Gut Connection: A Microbial Influence

The gut microbiome, the diverse community of microorganisms residing in the intestines, plays a pivotal role in the gut-brain axis. These microbial inhabitants communicate with the gut and brain through a variety of mechanisms, including the production of neurotransmitters, hormones, and inflammatory mediators.

A healthy gut microbiome contributes to a balanced immune system, reducing inflammation and promoting overall well-being. However, disruptions in the gut microbiome, known as dysbiosis, can lead to inflammation, increased intestinal permeability, and altered communication between the gut, brain, and immune system.

The Neuroendocrine-Immune System: A Hormonal Dialogue

The neuroendocrine-immune system (NIS) represents another bidirectional communication pathway, connecting the nervous, endocrine, and immune systems. The HPA axis, the primary stress response pathway, serves as a central component of the NIS.

When stress arises, the brain triggers the release of corticotropin-releasing hormone (CRH), which stimulates the adrenal glands to produce cortisol, the stress hormone. Cortisol, in turn, influences immune cell activity and modulates the inflammatory response.

The NIS also includes bidirectional connections between the nervous system and the immune system.

For instance, certain immune cells can release neurotransmitters, influencing brain function and behavior.

<u>Bidirectional Communication: Implications for Health and Disease</u>

The intricate interplay of bidirectional communication pathways underscores the interconnectedness of body systems and their profound impact on overall health and well-being. Disruptions in these pathways can contribute to various health conditions, including:

- Inflammatory bowel disease (IBD): Alterations in the gut microbiome and dysregulated immune responses play a role in IBD.

- Irritable bowel syndrome (IBS): Bidirectional communication imbalances between the gut and brain contribute to IBS symptoms.

- Autoimmune diseases: Disrupted immune regulation and communication between the gut, brain, and immune system are implicated in autoimmune diseases.

Understanding and Harnessing Bidirectional Communication

As research continues to unravel the complexities of bidirectional communication pathways, new therapeutic approaches are emerging. By targeting these pathways, we can potentially modulate gut-brain interactions, enhance immune function, and improve overall health outcomes.

Dietary interventions, stress management techniques, and probiotic supplementation are examples of strategies that can influence bidirectional communication pathways, promoting a healthy gut-brain connection and supporting overall well-being.

- Psychoneuroimmunology: The Science of the Mind-Body Connection

Psychoneuroimmunology (PNI) stands at the forefront of scientific exploration, unraveling the intricate web that connects the mind, nervous system, and immune response. This chapter delves into the rich landscape of PNI, shedding light on how emotions, thoughts, and mental states can profoundly influence the body's immune function.

Defining Psychoneuroimmunology

We commence by defining PNI, elucidating its roots in psychology, neuroscience, and immunology. Readers gain a nuanced understanding of how this interdisciplinary science seeks to decipher the bidirectional communication between the brain, nervous system, and immune system.

The Impact of Stress on Immunity

A focal point of the chapter is the exploration of stress and its effects on the immune system. We delve into groundbreaking studies that unveil the intricate mechanisms through which chronic stress can compromise immune function. From cortisol release to alterations in immune cell activity, readers gain insights into the physiological toll of stress on the body.

Emotions and Immune Responses

Building on stress, we examine how a spectrum of emotions, from joy to sadness, can shape immune responses. PNI research has uncovered how positive emotions can enhance immune function, while negative emotions may contribute to susceptibility to illness. Real-life examples and case studies provide tangible illustrations of these connections.

Neural Pathways of Influence

To deepen understanding, we explore the neural pathways that serve as conduits between the brain and the immune system. Discussions on the role of neurotransmitters, such as serotonin and dopamine, reveal how these chemical messengers mediate the cross-talk between mental processes and immune activity.

Mind-Body Interventions

The chapter transitions into the practical realm by discussing mind-body interventions that harness PNI principles for health benefits. From meditation and mindfulness to yoga and biofeedback, we showcase how these practices can positively impact both mental well-being and immune function.

Individual Variability and Resilience

Acknowledging the diversity of individual responses, we discuss how genetics, environment, and lifestyle contribute to variability in psychoneuroimmunological outcomes. Highlighting the concept of resilience, we explore factors that can bolster an individual's ability to navigate stressors without compromising immune health.

Future Avenues in PNI Research

Concluding the chapter, we glimpse into the future of PNI. Emerging research avenues, technological advancements, and the potential for personalized interventions underscore the ongoing evolution of this field, leaving readers with a sense of the dynamic nature of mind-body research.

This exploration of psychoneuroimmunology serves to demystify the profound connections between mental states and immune responses, empowering readers to appreciate the science behind the mind-body connection and consider its implications for their own well-being.

Chapter 7. How Diet and Lifestyle Influence Mental and Physical Health

- Effects of Exercise on the Mind and Body

Exercise is a powerful tool that can improve your physical and mental health in many ways. It can help you lose weight, build muscle, and improve your cardiovascular health. It can also help you reduce stress, anxiety, and depression.

<u>Physical Benefits of Exercise</u>

Weight loss: Exercise can help you lose weight by burning calories and increasing your metabolism.

Muscle building: Exercise can help you build muscle by increasing muscle mass and strength.

Improved cardiovascular health: Exercise can help improve your cardiovascular health by lowering your blood pressure, cholesterol levels, and risk of heart disease.

Reduced risk of chronic diseases: Exercise can help reduce your risk of developing chronic diseases such as type 2 diabetes, stroke, and some types of cancer.

Stronger bones: Exercise can help you build stronger bones, which can help reduce your risk of osteoporosis.

Improved flexibility: Exercise can help improve your flexibility, which can help reduce your risk of injury.

Mental Benefits of Exercise

Reduced stress: Exercise can help reduce stress by releasing endorphins, which have mood-boosting effects.

Reduced anxiety: Exercise can help reduce anxiety by distracting you from your worries and helping you to focus on the present moment.

Reduced depression: Exercise can help reduce depression by improving your mood and self-esteem.

Improved sleep: Exercise can help you sleep better by tiring you out physically and mentally.

Increased energy: Exercise can help you increase your energy levels by improving your circulation and oxygen intake.

Improved cognitive function: Exercise can help improve your cognitive function by increasing blood flow to the brain and stimulating the growth of new brain cells.

How Much Physical Activity Is Enough?

Adults should engage in at least 150 minutes of moderate-intensity aerobic activity or 75 minutes of vigorous-intensity aerobic activity every week, according to the Centers for Disease Control and Prevention (CDC). Adults should also engage in muscle-strengthening activities that target all main muscle groups (legs, hips, back, belly, chest, shoulders, and arms) at least twice a week.

- Circadian Rhythms and Sleep

Sleep and circadian rhythms are critical components of the mind-gut immunological link. The host's circadian rhythms and the gut microbiome are interrelated, and changes in sleep and circadian rhythms can affect the gut microbiota, immunological function, and general health.

According to research, the gut microbiome has its own circadian rhythm, and changes in gut microbiome populations over time are crucial for general health. The gut microbiota controls not just the metabolic response to nutrition, but also the host's sleep and mental moods. Preliminary data suggests that bacteria and circadian genes can interact, and that the gut microbiome and metabolism are linked to the host's circadian rhythms.

Changes in gut microbial diversity and composition have been related to sleep deprivation and circadian misalignment. Inadequate sleep and circadian misalignment are linked to poor metabolic health outcomes, and changes in gut microbial diversity and composition may be one mechanism by which sleep and circadian rhythms influence metabolic health.

Sleep, circadian rhythms, and the gut flora all have a bidirectional link. The gut microbiota can influence sleep and circadian rhythms, and the gut microbiome can influence sleep and circadian rhythms. Interfering with mice's sleep patterns can modify the structure and diversity of their gut microbiota, and circadian clock misalignment, sleep deprivation, and

shift work can impact circadian clock gene
expression and the structure of their microbial
communities.

Chapter 8: Healthy Mind, Gut, and Immune System Strategies

- Stress Reduction Techniques

Both external and internal factors contribute to stress. External influences include your physical surroundings, employment, interpersonal interactions, house, and all of the problems, challenges, difficulties, and expectations you face on a regular basis.

Internal variables influence your body's capacity to respond to and deal with external stressors. Your dietary condition, general health and fitness levels, emotional well-being, capacity to reduce stress through relaxation techniques or other measures, and quantity of sleep and rest you get are all internal aspects that impact your ability to handle stress.

Managing stress might thus entail acquiring techniques to modify the external circumstances that face you or internal aspects that increase your ability to deal with whatever comes your way. The following are five major stress-relieving techniques:

Exercise

Meditation and relaxation approaches

Time management

Organizational abilities

Systems of assistance

Yoga

Through a variety of postural and breathing techniques, one purpose of yoga is to restore balance and harmony to the body and emotions.

Structured relaxation techniques may be used in a variety of ways to help regulate stress and enhance your physical and emotional well-being. While some forms of meditation and relaxation therapies are best learnt in a class setting, meditation methods may also be learned on your own. There are several relaxation methods available, ranging from audio CDs to group martial arts and fitness sessions.

The following are only a few examples of organized programs that might boost our capacity for relaxation:

Autogenic training is a technique that was developed in the early twentieth century and is focused on passive attention and awareness of bodily sensations. The repeating of so-called autogenic "formulas" concentrates attention on distinct feelings, such as warmth or heaviness, in different parts of the body. Physicians have employed autogenic training as part of therapy for a variety of illnesses. Popular in Europe (and even covered by certain insurance plans), this practice is now gaining traction in the United States. There are no specific physical talents or exercises required; nonetheless, anyone interested in learning this approach must be willing to spend time and patience. Because this technique is significantly more sophisticated than some relaxation methods, taking a course is usually the best way to learn it.

Biofeedback is one approach of learning to relax, control stress responses, or adjust the body's reactions by using monitoring equipment that delivers information from the body that would otherwise be unavailable. This strategy is based on the notion, initially proposed in the early 1960s, that the autonomic nervous system (the portion of our nervous system that we do not consciously utilize) is trainable. For example, when people experiment with posture modifications, breathing methods, or thinking patterns, equipment can be used to monitor heart rate, blood pressure, brain activity, stomach acidity, muscular tension, or other parameters. Receiving this input allows one to learn to identify the processes that result in the desired outcome, such as a decrease in heart rate and blood pressure. Many practitioners utilize biofeedback to treat a wide range of psychological and physical disorders. The procedure can only be conducted by a professional because it requires the use of measurement instruments.

Imagery, often known as guided imagery, is the use of pleasant or calming pictures to quiet the mind and body. Deep relaxation can be achieved by regulating breathing and imagining a calming image. This strategy may be learnt by anybody and is simple to implement.

Meditation approaches: Meditation is one of the most common strategies for achieving physical and mental relaxation. It ranges from activities connected with certain faiths or beliefs to methods concentrating only on physical relaxation. There are thousands of distinct styles of meditation, and many of them are self-learning. The meditative state is one of profound concentration and focusing on one's fundamental being; there is a quieting of the mind, emotions, and body. The meditative state can be attained through scheduled (as in a regular routine) or unstructured (as in being alone outdoors) activities. While there are many teachers of contemplative arts accessible, certain methods may be learnt through books or internet tutorials.

Transcendental meditation (TM) is a type of meditation that has been popular for several decades. The purpose of TM is to achieve transcendental consciousness (the most basic kind of awareness). It is quite straightforward to learn and is practiced for 15-20 minutes in the mornings and nights. For novices, there are several programs and educational materials accessible.

Another meditation approach has grown in popularity in the United States since its description in the 1970s by Harvard physician Herbert Benson. This approach includes producing the so-called relaxation response by repeating a word or phrase while sitting quietly for 10-20 minutes every day. This strategy has no religious or spiritual undertones and is designed to elicit the opposite physical reaction to the stress response (or "fight or flight" reflex). Its effectiveness has been demonstrated in lowering blood pressure and other physical stress reactions. It, like other types of meditation, may be mastered on one's own, but it takes time and effort to achieve the desired level of calm.

Progressive muscle relaxation is a technique established in the 1930s in which muscle groups are contracted and then released in sequence. This strategy is founded on the assumption that mental relaxation will occur as a natural result of physical relaxation. Although there is some muscle movement involved, this method does not need any specific abilities or fitness and can be mastered by virtually anybody. Progressive muscular relaxation is usually done for 10-20 minutes each day. For greatest effects, as with the relaxation response, practice and patience are necessary.

Qigong: Qigong is a martial art that blends physical training (such as isometrics, isotonic, and aerobic conditioning) with Eastern philosophy and relaxation methods. There are several types of qigong, including medical qigong. Some types are performed standing, sitting, or lying down, while others include regulated motions or massage. Over 70 million Chinese people practice some type of qigong every day. Qigong has been utilized in China for generations to treat a wide range of medical issues. Learning qigong takes time, effort, patience, and persistence, and it is best to learn from a master or group. Because this procedure requires physical exertion, see your doctor before commencing, especially if you have a chronic medical condition or are over the age of 40.

Tai chi is a Chinese martial technique similar to qigong. It has been described as "meditation in motion" because of its gentle, flowing motions that emphasize accuracy and energy. This practice, also known as tai chi chuan, dates back thousands of years. Training from a master, like with qigong, is required to acquire the technique of tai chi. Again, because motion and power are necessary, consult your doctor before starting training.

Yoga is an ancient Indian type of exercise that is founded on the notion that the body and breathing are linked with the mind. Yoga is said to have been practiced for over 5,000 years. Through a variety of postural and breathing techniques, one purpose of yoga is to restore balance and harmony to the body and emotions. Yoga, which means "joining" or "union" in Sanskrit, has been described as the "search for the soul" and the "union between the individual and the divine." Yoga advantages include greater flexibility and relaxation capability. Yoga does not require any specific conditioning and may be learnt by almost anyone. There are several classes, books, and videos accessible. Those with unique or chronic physical issues should see their doctor before commencing.

Time management and organizing abilities are required.

Effective stress management requires good time management abilities. Learning to prioritize work and avoid overcommitting are two key methods to avoid being overscheduled. Using a calendar or planner consistently and checking it before committing to anything is one approach to improve time management abilities. You may also learn to identify time-wasting jobs by maintaining a diary for a few days and seeing where you could be squandering time.

Instead than becoming a slave to incoming information, productivity gurus advocate setting up a certain time (or numerous times) each day to check and reply to email and texts. Another time management skill that may be learnt or improved is the ability to avoid procrastination.

You won't have to deal with the stress of misplaced goods and clutter if your physical surroundings (office, desk, kitchen, closet, and automobile) are neatly organized. Make it a practice to clean out and go through the piles of paperwork and clutter that build up over time.

Systems of assistance

People with strong social support systems have less physical and mental stress symptoms than those who are less connected. Our social networks include loved ones, friends, professional partners, neighbors, and even pets. Creating and maintaining a social support network is beneficial to both the body and the mind.

Strategies to obtain Stress Management

If you believe you are unable to cope with or manage stress on your own, or if you are experiencing excruciating stress, remember that there are tools available to assist you.

Consult with your doctor. Stress may have a negative impact on your health, making you more susceptible to infections and exacerbating the symptoms of almost any chronic disease. Stress can also produce a variety of physical problems. Your doctor will be able to analyze the impact of stress on your physical functioning and will be able to offer measures to resist these negative consequences. Remember to be open and honest about your level of stress. In extreme situations of short-term life stress, your doctor might discuss pharmaceutical options with you to assist ease the symptoms. He or she can also recommend relaxation methods and advise you on the best stress-reduction measures for you. If you decide to consult a counselor or therapist, your doctor is a great place to start.

Consider getting therapy. Various sorts of mental-health experts provide stress-management therapy. Stress counseling and group discussion therapy have been shown to help reduce stress symptoms and enhance overall health and attitude. Counseling does not have to be a long-term commitment, but for some people, a series of stress-reduction sessions with a trained therapist will be beneficial. He or she can assist you in identifying trouble areas in your life and developing techniques to manage your most stressful occasions or scenarios. Talking to an objective and sympathetic observer may also be a terrific method to release stress and concern.

Spend time with the people you care about. Numerous studies suggest that persons who have a healthy, joyful social support network (friends, family, loved ones, or even pets) have less stress-related symptoms and are better stress managers than those who do not have social support. Your loved ones are also in an ideal position to watch your lifestyle and give advice and assistance when necessary.

Take a class. Many relaxation programs, meditation techniques, and approaches for mental and physical relaxation are essentially taught processes that are best studied in a class or course with an experienced instructor. Another advantage is that you will meet others who share your aims and hobbies.

Adults are also affected by ADHD.

ADHD is not just a childhood illness; 30% to 70% of children with ADHD continue to have symptoms as they grow older. Furthermore, persons who were never identified as children may have more evident symptoms as adults, causing problems at work or in relationships. Many individuals are unaware that they have ADHD, leaving them perplexed as to why their ambitions appear to elude them.

Adult ADHD Symptoms: Being Late

ADHD manifests itself in adults in a somewhat different way than it does in children. Adults may consistently be late for work or crucial events. Adults may recognize that their tardiness is jeopardizing their ambitions, but they just can't seem to get things done on time.

Adult ADHD Symptoms: Dangerous Driving

One of the characteristics of ADHD is trouble focusing your attention on the work at hand. When kids and adults get behind the wheel of a car, this spells disaster. According to studies, persons with ADHD are more likely to speed, get into accidents, and lose their driver's license.

Adult ADHD Symptoms: Distraction

Adults with ADHD may struggle with task prioritization, starting, and completion. They are unorganized, agitated, and easily distracted. Some persons with ADHD struggle to concentrate when reading. Inability to focus and complete activities may jeopardize jobs, goals, and relationships.

Adult ADHD Symptoms: Outbursts

Adults with ADHD may struggle with self-control. This can result in:

Controlling rage is difficult.

impulsive actions

expressing harsh or offensive sentiments

ADHD Symptoms

Adult ADHD Symptoms: Hyperfocus

Some individuals with ADHD have the ability to hyperfocus on topics they love or find intriguing. However, they struggle to focus on jobs that boring them. The problem is that many chores required for success in everyday life, from preparing a grocery list to filing paperwork at work, are tedious. People with ADHD prefer to put off unpleasant chores in favor of more pleasurable ones.

What Are the Causes of ADHD?

Neurotransmitters, which are brain chemicals, are less active in parts of the brain that affect attention in patients with ADHD. Researchers are unsure what causes this chemical imbalance, but they believe genes may play a part because ADHD frequently runs in families. Prenatal exposure to smokes and alcohol has also been associated to ADHD in studies.

ADHD Diagnosis in Adults

Many individuals might not realize they have ADHD until they seek treatment for another issue, such as anxiety or depression. Discussing bad behaviors, problems at work, or marital problems frequently indicates that ADHD is to blame. To be confirmed, the condition must have existed during childhood, even if it was never identified. Childhood issues such as poor attention and hyperactivity can be documented using old report cards or by speaking with family.

Some mental health practitioners employ neuropsychological testing during an ADHD examination. Timed, computer-based assessments that assess attention and problem-solving abilities are examples of this. Although neuropsychological testing is not required to obtain a diagnosis, it can provide insight into how ADHD impacts a person's everyday life. It can also detect comorbid problems like learning impairments.

ADHD Complications in Adults

Coping with adult ADHD symptoms may be exhausting in and of itself. Simultaneously, many individuals with ADHD suffer from despair, anxiety, or obsessive compulsive disorder. They are also more prone to smoke or use illegal substances. People with ADHD can mitigate these issues by obtaining appropriate therapy.

Treatments for ADHD

Stimulants are the most commonly prescribed medications for ADHD. It may appear paradoxical that stimulants are used to aid persons who are restless or hyperactive. By fine-tuning brain circuitry that impact attention, these medicines may improve focus and reduce distractibility. If stimulants are ineffective, your doctor may prescribe an antidepressant or a selective norepinephrine reuptake inhibitor, such as atomoxetine, to assist manage impulsive behaviors.

Chapter 9: The Beneficial Effects of Probiotics on Mental Health

- Knowledge of Probiotics and Prebiotics

Prebiotics are chemicals that are indigestible by the human GI tract (resistant to secretions and intestinal enzymes) and pass through the gut intact to reach the colon. The gut microbiome (GM) or probiotic bacteria that are fed together break down prebiotics in the colon to create beneficial chemicals. Indeed, prebiotic breakdown not only generates therapeutic and health-promoting chemicals, but it also strengthens and functions colon-based probiotics as a food supply. Carbohydrates and the families of galactooligosaccharides (GOS), fructooligosaccharides (FOS), and xylooligosaccharides (XOS) are the most significant prebiotics (2). According to the National Health and

Nutrition Examination Survey (NHANES), people over the age of 20 in the United States consume only 61% of their recommended level of prebiotics. While there is no official data on prebiotic consumption, researchers recommend consuming 10 g of FOS or 7 g of GOS per day (9, 10). Prebiotics work in small quantities; for example, polydextrose has an effective quantity of 2 to 7.5 g per day (11), resistant starch has an effective amount of 2.5 to 5 g per day (12), and inulin has an effective amount of 1 to 6 g per day (13).

Synbiotics, which mix probiotics and prebiotics, have a synergistic impact and play an essential role in managing and lowering the risk of certain diseases, including mental disorders. The amount of probiotics reduces in the absence of prebiotics, which are regarded a food source for probiotics, producing difficulties with the host's intestinal and general immune systems, as well as certain irregularities such as constipation. Prebiotics, on the other hand, will have a smaller function in host health and disease management if there are no probiotics or their quantity is very low (14). Numerous studies have indicated that probiotics and prebiotics, whether taken together or separately, have a crucial role in neuroimmune processes. It has also been demonstrated that their CNS health benefits are connected to interactions between GM and colon-based probiotics, the immune, and neural systems, which occur through the release of certain enzymes, hormones, immunological factors, and neurotransmitters (5, 15, 16). Furthermore, animal, clinical, and paraclinical studies have revealed a link between the presence and activity of probiotics and prebiotics in the gut, CNS, and immune systems, and the incidence of Alzheimer's, depression, schizophrenia, anxiety, autism, insomnia, severe stress, and other mental diseases (5, 17).

This review discusses the prospective function of probiotics and prebiotics in regulating the immunological and neural systems, as well as the possible management and treatment of several mental diseases. These supplements' probable mechanisms of action in the healing process of CNS illnesses have also been explored. Finally, the study concludes with an outline of the future potential for employing these chemicals to treat mental diseases.

Mood Disorders and Probiotics

Background: Probiotics and their nutritional sources (prebiotics) have been demonstrated to have beneficial effects on many host organs. The concept of their potential benefits on the Central Nervous System (CNS) and the incidence of Anxiety, Schizophrenia, Alzheimer, Depression, Autism, and other mental disorders has proposed a new category of medicines called "psychobiotic" which is hoped to be of low-side effect anti-inflammatory, antidepressant, and anti-anxiety constituents.

The current review provides valuable insights into the complicated interactions between the GI microbiota (particularly in the colon), brain, immune, and central nervous systems, as well as a summary of the main findings of the effects of probiotics and prebiotics on important mental disorders, from potential mechanisms of action to clinical application.

Methods: The following key phrases were searched in Google Scholar, Pub Med, Scopus, and Science Direct databases: "probiotics", "prebiotics", "mental disorders", "psychological disorders", "depression", "anxiety", "stress", "Alzheimer", and "autism spectrum". The reviewers obtained and thoroughly evaluated the complete text of possibly qualifying papers. Data from the selected publications were retrieved and summarized.

The research suggests that probiotics and prebiotics may boost brain performance through a variety of methods. Clinical studies have also shown that its use can help with depression, anxiety, Alzheimer's disease, and autistic spectrum disorders.

Conclusion: Probiotics and prebiotics can improve mental health and psychological function and could be used as new medicines for common mental disorders; however, more clinical research is needed to determine the clinical significance of the effects and their bioequivalence or superiority to current treatments.

- Clinical Use of Probiotics

The discovery that gut bacterial microflora might modify immune system surveillance via altered dietary choices has increased awareness of the importance of probiotics. These are living microorganisms that may enter the gastrointestinal system and modify its microfloral makeup, resulting in favorable health benefits when taken in sufficient quantities. Probiotics' clinical usefulness in the treatment and prevention of a wide range of acute and chronic gastrointestinal disorders, as well as non-gastrointestinal diseases such as atopy, respiratory infections, vaginitis, and hypercholesterolaemia, has been studied in recent clinical trials. Because the microbes in probiotic supplements are comparable to those found in human gastrointestinal and vaginal microbiota, they are widely recognized as harmless. Guidelines for the use of probiotics in the clinical arena necessitate regular changes in order for the most recent evidence to be included in clinical applications. The goal of this clinical report is to examine the most recent research on the use of probiotics in a variety of gastrointestinal and non-gastrointestinal disorders.

Chapter 10: The Role of Antioxidants in Promoting Mental and Gut Health

Inflammation and Oxidative Stress

The mind-gut immunological link is dependent on oxidative stress and inflammation. Oxidative stress arises when there is an imbalance between the formation of reactive oxygen species (ROS) and the ability of the protective system to detoxify these reactive products. It can harm cells and tissues and create persistent inflammation. Long-term oxidative stress can also lead to diabetes, cancer, and heart disease. The normal immune response can generate oxidative stress, which can contribute to mild inflammation. It fades gone as the body's immunity to the virus is strengthened. Uncontrolled oxidative stress can hasten the aging process and contribute to a variety of additional problems. Food/diet, lifestyle, and environmental variables such as pollution and radiation all contribute to oxidative stress. Antioxidant-rich foods for lowering oxidative stress include spinach, pumpkin, pecans, beetroot, collard greens, cabbage, berries, broccoli, carrots, avocados, and sweet potatoes.

Inflammation is the process by which your body works to repair itself after being infected, sick, or injured. The immune system produces it as a typical reaction to these situations. Chronic inflammation, on the other hand, can lead to a variety of health issues, including heart disease, diabetes, and cancer. Chronic inflammation can be caused by oxidative stress. Infections and injuries activate the immune system. While fighting off invading bacteria, immune cells called macrophages create free radicals. These free radicals can cause inflammation by causing harm to healthy cells. In most cases, inflammation subsides when the immune system has eliminated the infection or repaired the injured tissue. However, oxidative stress may also cause an inflammatory response, which creates more free radicals, which can lead to further oxidative stress, creating a vicious cycle.

Diabetes, cardiovascular disease, and arthritis can all be caused by chronic inflammation caused by oxidative stress. The consequences of oxidative stress may have a role in the development of numerous neurodegenerative diseases, including Alzheimer's and Parkinson's. It has been demonstrated that oxidative stress increases redox signaling, transcription factor activation, the activity of pro-inflammatory and pro-fibrotic cascades, DNA damage, and the induction of stress-dependent kinases. Furthermore, immune cells employ large ROS production (oxidative burst) to eliminate invading infections. The relationship between pro-inflammatory cytokine signaling and oxidative stress is being investigated. Overexpression of pro-inflammatory cytokines, for example, has been found to promote ROS production.

- Food Antioxidants

Antioxidants are food-derived substances that scavenge and neutralize free radicals, which are unstable molecules that can harm cell membranes and other bodily components. Free radicals are formed in the human body during the oxidation process, which happens when oxygen is metabolized. The body can deal with certain free radicals and need them to operate properly, but an excess of free radicals over time can produce oxidative stress, which can cause cell and tissue damage and chronic inflammation. Diabetes, cancer, and heart disease are among illnesses that can be caused by oxidative stress.

Certain foods, including as fruits and vegetables, nuts, whole grains, and some meats, contain antioxidants. Plant foods are particularly high in antioxidants. Vitamins A, C, and E, as well as the minerals copper, zinc, and selenium, are nutritional antioxidants that can help prevent free radical damage by neutralizing it. Antioxidant pills, according to evidence, do not work as effectively as naturally occurring antioxidants in diets.

The gut-brain axis is a two-way communication system that connects the central nervous system to the enteric nervous system, which includes the digestive tract. Recent study has revealed that probiotics and prebiotics can affect the gut-brain axis, which benefits the central nervous system and lowers the risk of mental health issues. Probiotics are live microorganisms that have one or more positive effects on the host when consumed in appropriate numbers. Prebiotics are chemicals that are indigestible by the human digestive tract but serve as a nutrition source for probiotics that settle non the colon.

Several studies have found that probiotics and prebiotics can improve mental health, including mood and cognitive performance. According to several studies, probiotics may assist improve mood and cognitive performance, as well as reduce stress and anxiety. For example, one study discovered that Alzheimer's patients who received milk containing four probiotic bacteria species for 12 weeks performed better on a cognitive impairment test than those who consumed ordinary milk.

- Supplementation with antioxidants

The possible influence of antioxidant supplementation on the mind-gut immunological link is a topic of considerable attention in the realm of nutrition. Antioxidants are substances that can aid in the neutralization of free radicals, which are unstable chemicals that can cause cell damage and contribute to oxidative stress and inflammation. Oxidative stress and inflammation are important components of the mind-gut immunological system and can have serious consequences for both mental and physical health.

Antioxidants may be present in a wide range of foods, including fruits and vegetables, nuts, and whole grains. They are found in high concentrations in plant foods and are particularly high in vitamins A, C, and E, as well as the minerals copper, zinc, and selenium. Antioxidant supplements are also available and are frequently advertised as a means of strengthening the body's defenses against oxidative stress and inflammation.

So far, the studies have been ambiguous, but they do not give solid evidence that antioxidant supplements have a significant influence on illness. Remember that the effect of antioxidant supplements on illness is yet unknown, and more study is required to properly understand their potential benefits and hazards. While some studies have shown that antioxidant supplements may have a good influence on mental and physical health, others have found no meaningful benefit.

Chapter 11. Stress Reduction Techniques for a Healthy Mind and Body

Cognitive Behavioral Therapy (CBT)

Cognitive Behavioral Therapy (CBT) is a type of psychological treatment that has been shown to be useful for a variety of issues such as depression, anxiety disorders, alcohol and drug use issues, marital problems, eating disorders, and serious mental disease. CBT focuses on modifying the automatic negative beliefs that can contribute to and aggravate emotional disorders, and it has been demonstrated to enhance functioning and quality of life significantly. CBT is based on several core principles, including the notion that psychological problems are, in part, caused by faulty or unhelpful ways of thinking, and that people suffering from psychological problems can learn better ways of

coping with them, relieving their symptoms and becoming more effective in their lives.

CBT treatment often entails efforts to modify thought patterns, and these tactics may include learning to notice one's own thinking distortions that are causing issues and then reevaluating them in light of reality, as well as learning to quiet one's mind and relax one's body. CBT focuses on teaching people how to be their own therapists, and patients are assisted to build coping skills through exercises in the session as well as "homework" tasks outside of sessions. CBT is a prominent sort of organized talk therapy (psychotherapy) that helps individuals become aware of erroneous or negative thinking so they may perceive challenging events more clearly and respond to them more effectively. CBT may be a highly beneficial technique in treating mental health illnesses such as depression, PTSD, or an eating disorder, and it can also be used to assist anybody learn how to better manage stressful life events.

- Neurofeedback and biofeedback

Biofeedback and neurofeedback are procedures that can help people learn to manage their physiological reactions to stress and enhance their general well-being. Biofeedback is a sort of mind-body treatment in which physiological processes such as heart rate, muscular tension, and skin temperature are measured and feedback is provided. Neurofeedback is a sort of biofeedback that measures and provides feedback on brainwave activity via electronic monitoring. Both strategies may be used to teach people how to manage their physiological reactions to stress and enhance their general well-being.

Biofeedback and neurofeedback are founded on the idea that by being more aware of their physiological processes and learning to manage them, people may learn to control their physiological reactions to stress and enhance their general well-being. Biofeedback, for example, may be used to teach people how to manage their heart rate and muscle tension, whereas neurofeedback can teach people how to control their brainwave activity. Both strategies can help people learn to relax and lower their overall stress levels.

Biofeedback and neurofeedback have been demonstrated to help with a variety of issues, including anxiety, depression, chronic pain, and sleeplessness. Biofeedback, for example, has been proven to reduce muscular tension and improve general relaxation, whilst neurofeedback has been demonstrated to reduce anxiety and improve overall well-being. Both strategies may be used to teach people how to relax and lower their overall stress levels, which can improve their general well-being.

Chapter 12: Sleep Hygiene: Making Rest a Priority for a Healthy Mind and Immune System

- The Sleep Science

Michel Gondry's 2006 surrealistic scientific fantasy comedy film "The Science of Sleep" was written and directed by him. The film, starring Gael Garcia Bernal, delves into the whimsical and dreamy aspect of sleep and the human psyche. However, for the sake of "The Mind-Gut Immune Connection" book, we shall concentrate on the scientific features of sleep and their relation to the mind-gut immune link.

Sleep is a crucial physiological activity for general health and well-being. It is a complex and dynamic condition defined by fluctuations in brain wave activity, heart rate, breathing rate, and body temperature. Non-rapid eye movement (NREM) sleep and rapid eye movement (REM) sleep are the two basic phases of sleep. NREM sleep is further subdivided into three phases, each corresponding to a deeper degree of sleep.

Sleep research is a fast developing area that has achieved substantial improvements in our knowledge of the physiological and psychological processes that occur during sleep. Sleep has been demonstrated in studies to play an important part in the regulation of the immune system, and sleep deprivation can have a deleterious influence on immunological function. Sleep is also necessary for memory consolidation, mood management, and emotional well-being.

The mind-gut immune link is a two-way communication mechanism that exists between the central nervous system, the enteric nervous system, and the immune system. Sleep plays an important role in the regulation of the mind-gut immunological relationship, and sleep deprivation can have a deleterious influence on gut health and immune function, according to research. Sleep is also necessary for the management of the gut microbiota, which is important in the mind-gut immunological link.

Chapter 13: Hydration and Its Effects on Mental and Physical Health

- Water and Cognitive Function

Water is required for brain function, and dehydration can impair cognitive ability and general brain health. Water is required for the creation of neurotransmitters and hormones, the regulation of fluid levels that protect the brain and spinal cord from stress and damage, and the clearance of toxins and metabolic waste that collect in the brain. According to research, even slight dehydration can result in a decline in cognitive function, including memory loss, poor concentration and attention, delayed information processing, irritability, and headaches. Drinking water has also been proven in studies to boost reaction speed while decreasing confusion and tension. Dehydration can impair psychological well-being and mood, in addition to impairing cognitive performance, because the body requires water to produce hormones and neurotransmitters like dopamine and serotonin, which regulate mood, and to ensure the proper functioning of these neurotransmitters and chemical processes. In conclusion, water is necessary for brain function, and dehydration can negatively impair cognitive performance and general brain health. It is critical to be hydrated in order to support and improve learning, thinking, attention, and overall brain function.

- Electrolyte Stability

Electrolyte balance is essential for the mind-gut immunological relationship because it promotes optimal gut and immune system function. Electrolytes are minerals that carry an electric charge and are necessary for many human activities, including adequate hydration, neuron and muscle function regulation, and pH balance. Sodium, potassium, chloride, calcium, magnesium, and phosphate are the most common electrolytes.

The ability of the gut's immune cells to protect against hazardous invaders is dependent on proper electrolyte balance. The stomach actively transfers electrolytes across its lining, influencing food absorption and maintaining the acidic environment necessary for digesting and fending off dangerous microorganisms. Sodium and potassium, in particular, play an important role in managing fluid equilibrium in the stomach, which is necessary for appropriate digestion and food passage through the digestive system. Electrolytes also serve to modulate nerve impulses in the stomach, controlling how the digestive system functions and ensuring that food travels through the gut at the proper rate, preventing constipation and diarrhea.

During heavy endurance exercise, the gut microbiota is linked to adequate hydration and electrolyte balance. Certain gut bacteria regulate cellular transit of electrolytes through the gut wall mucosa, and active electrogenic chlorine (electrolyte) release in the gut wall mucosa enhances the abundance of particular bacterial genera. The gut microbiota also helps to avoid excessive inflammatory reactions, which may be detrimental to the gut.

Chapter 14: Adopting a Balanced Diet for a Strong Mind, Gut, and Immune System

- The Mediterranean Diet

The Mediterranean diet is renowned for its health benefits, particularly for the mind, gut, and immune system. This diet emphasizes whole, unprocessed foods, and is rich in fruits, vegetables, whole grains, legumes, and healthy fats, such as olive oil and nuts. Here are seven Mediterranean diet principles to adopt for a balanced diet that supports a strong mind, gut, and immune system, along with ingredients and their preparation methods:

1. Emphasize Plant-Based Foods: The Mediterranean diet is centered around plant-based foods, including

fruits, vegetables, whole grains, legumes, and nuts. These foods are rich in fiber, vitamins, minerals, and antioxidants, which support a healthy gut and immune system.

- - Ingredients: Spinach, kale, tomatoes, bell peppers, zucchini, eggplant, artichokes, chickpeas, lentils, quinoa, brown rice, almonds, walnuts, and seeds.
- - Preparation Methods: Incorporate these ingredients into salads, soups, stews, and grain bowls. Use olive oil, lemon juice, and herbs for dressing.

2. Include Fatty Fish and Lean Protein: Fatty fish, such as salmon, sardines, and mackerel, are rich in omega-3 fatty acids, which support brain health and reduce inflammation. Lean protein sources, such as poultry, eggs, and legumes, provide essential amino acids for overall health.

- - Ingredients: Salmon, sardines, mackerel, chicken, turkey, eggs, and legumes.

- - preparation Methods: Grill or bake fish with herbs and lemon. Prepare lean protein with herbs, garlic, and olive oil. Include eggs in omelets, frittatas, or as a protein source in salads.

3. Healthy Fats: The Mediterranean diet is abundant in healthy fats, particularly from extra virgin olive oil, nuts, and seeds. These fats support brain health, reduce inflammation, and aid in nutrient absorption.

- Ingredients: Extra virgin olive oil, olives, avocados, almonds, walnuts, and seeds.
- Preparation Methods: Use extra virgin olive oil for cooking, salad dressings, and dips. Snack on a handful of nuts or seeds. Add avocado to salads, sandwiches, or smoothies.

4. Herbs and Spices: Herbs and spices not only enhance the flavor of dishes but also provide antioxidants and anti-inflammatory compounds that support overall health.

- Ingredients: Basil, oregano, rosemary, thyme, mint, parsley, garlic, and turmeric.
- Preparation Methods: Use herbs and spices to season dishes, soups, and sauces. Create herb-infused olive oils or vinegars for added flavor.

5. Whole Grains: Whole grains, such as quinoa, brown rice, and whole grain bread, provide fiber, vitamins, and minerals that support a healthy gut and immune system.

- Ingredients: Quinoa, brown rice, whole grain bread, barley, and farro.
- Preparation Methods: Use whole grains as a base for grain bowls, salads, or side dishes. Prepare whole grain bread for sandwiches or toast.

6. Fruits and Vegetables: Fruits and vegetables are rich in fiber, vitamins, minerals, and antioxidants that support a healthy gut and immune system.

- **- Ingredients: Berries, citrus fruits, apples, pears, leafy greens, broccoli, carrots, and bell peppers.**
- **- Preparation Methods: Enjoy fruits as snacks, in smoothies, or as a topping for yogurt. Incorporate vegetables into salads, stir-fries, and side dishes.**

7. Moderate Red Wine Consumption: Red wine, when consumed in moderation, provides antioxidants, such as resveratrol, that support heart health and reduce inflammation.

- **- Ingredients: Red wine (in moderation).**
- **- Preparation Methods: Enjoy a glass of red wine with meals as part of a balanced diet.**

Incorporating these Mediterranean diet principles into your daily routine can support a strong mind, gut, and immune system, while also providing a variety of delicious and nutritious meals.

- Plant-Based Diets

A plant-based diet is a nutrient-dense and fiber-rich diet that emphasizes whole, unprocessed foods, including fruits, vegetables, whole grains, legumes, nuts, and seeds. Adopting a plant-based diet can support a strong mind, gut, and immune system by providing essential nutrients, antioxidants, and anti-inflammatory compounds. Here are seven plant-based diets to adopt for a balanced diet that supports a strong mind, gut, and immune system, along with ingredients and their preparation methods:

1. Whole-Food, Plant-Based Diet: A whole-food, plant-based diet is based on natural, unprocessed, or minimally processed ingredients. This diet is free of animal ingredients such as meat, milk, eggs, or honey.

- - Ingredients: Fruits, vegetables, whole grains, legumes, nuts, and seeds.
- - Preparation Methods: Incorporate these ingredients into salads, soups, stews, and

grain bowls. Use olive oil, lemon juice, and herbs for dressing.

2. Mediterranean Diet: The Mediterranean diet emphasizes plant-based foods, including fruits, vegetables, whole grains, legumes, and healthy fats, such as olive oil and nuts.

- •   - Ingredients: Fruits, vegetables, whole grains, legumes, nuts, seeds, fatty fish, and lean protein sources.
- •   - Preparation Methods: Grill or bake fish with herbs and lemon. Prepare lean protein with herbs, garlic, and olive oil. Include eggs in omelets, frittatas, or as a protein source in salads.

3. Flexitarian Diet: The flexitarian diet is a plant-based diet that allows for occasional consumption of animal products.

- •   - Ingredients: Fruits, vegetables, whole grains, legumes, nuts, seeds, lean protein sources, and occasional animal products.

- - Preparation Methods: Incorporate these ingredients into salads, soups, stews, and grain bowls. Use olive oil, lemon juice, and herbs for dressing.

4. Vegetarian Diet: A vegetarian diet is free of meat, poultry, and fish, but may include dairy products and eggs.

- Ingredients: Fruits, vegetables, whole grains, legumes, nuts, seeds, dairy products, and eggs.
- Preparation Methods: Incorporate these ingredients into salads, soups, stews, and grain bowls. Use olive oil, lemon juice, and herbs for dressing.

5. Vegan Diet: A vegan diet is free of all animal products, including meat, poultry, fish, dairy products, and eggs.

- - Ingredients: Fruits, vegetables, whole grains, legumes, nuts, and seeds.

- - preparation Methods: Incorporate these ingredients into salads, soups, stews, and grain bowls. Use olive oil, lemon juice, and herbs for dressing.

6. Raw Food Diet: A raw food diet is based on uncooked or minimally cooked foods, including fruits, vegetables, nuts, and seeds.

- - Ingredients: Fruits, vegetables, nuts, and seeds.
- - Preparation Methods: Incorporate these ingredients into salads, smoothies, and raw desserts.

7. Macrobiotic Diet: A macrobiotic diet is based on whole, unprocessed foods, including whole grains, vegetables, legumes, and sea vegetables.

- - Ingredients: Whole grains, vegetables, legumes, sea vegetables, and occasional fish.
- - Preparation Methods: Incorporate these ingredients into soups, stews, and grain

bowls. Use miso, tamari, and seaweed for seasoning.

Incorporating these plant-based diets into your daily routine can support a strong mind, gut, and immune system, while also providing a variety of delicious and nutritious meals.

- Personalized Nutrition

1. Genetic Testing and Individualized Nutrient Needs: Genetic testing can provide insights into an individual's unique nutrient needs and potential health risks. Based on genetic information, personalized nutrition plans may include specific foods or supplements to support optimal health.

2. Food Sensitivity Testing and Personalized Elimination Diets: Food sensitivity testing can identify foods that may be causing inflammation or other adverse reactions in an individual's body. Based on food sensitivity testing results, personalized

nutrition plans may exclude certain foods or include alternatives to support optimal health.

3. Individualized Macronutrient Ratios and Meal Planning: Personalized nutrition plans may include specific macronutrient ratios, such as a higher protein or lower carbohydrate intake, based on an individual's unique needs. Meal planning and preparation strategies can also be tailored to support healthy eating habits.

4. Micronutrient Supplementation and Nutrient-Dense Foods: Personalized nutrition plans may include specific micronutrient supplements, such as vitamins or minerals, to support optimal health. Nutrient-dense foods can also be incorporated to meet individual nutrient needs.

5. Gut Health and Personalized Probiotic and Prebiotic Recommendations: Personalized nutrition plans may include specific probiotic and prebiotic recommendations to support gut health and the gut-brain axis. Fermented foods and high-fiber foods can also be included to support a healthy gut microbiome.

6. Mindful Eating and Stress Reduction Strategies: Personalized nutrition plans may include strategies for mindful eating, such as paying attention to hunger and fullness cues and avoiding distractions during meals. Stress reduction techniques and relaxation strategies can also be tailored to support overall well-being.

7. Lifestyle Modifications and Personalized Exercise Recommendations: Personalized nutrition plans may include lifestyle modifications, such as exercise recommendations, to support optimal health. Exercise plans can be tailored to an individual's unique needs and preferences.

Chapter 15: The Role of Exercise in Promoting Mental and Physical Well-being

- Types of Exercise and Their Benefits

Exercise plays a crucial role in maintaining overall health and well-being, including the mind-gut immune connection. There are various types of exercise, each with its own unique benefits. Here, we will discuss four main types of exercise and their benefits:

1. **Aerobic Exercise**: This type of exercise involves activities that increase the heart rate and breathing rate, typically over a prolonged period of time. Aerobic exercise has been shown to have a positive effect on both physical and mental well-being. It reduces the risk of various conditions such as cancer, diabetes, heart disease, stroke,

dementia, and other cognitive dysfunctions, while also reducing levels of inflammation in the body and, in moderation, improving immune system function.

2. **Resistance Training**: Resistance training involves the use of resistance to muscular contraction, such as weights or resistance bands. This type of exercise has been shown to improve muscle strength and endurance, as well as reduce the risk of osteoporosis, diabetes, and heart disease. Resistance training can also help improve cognitive function and reduce symptoms of depression and anxiety.

3. **Flexibility Exercise**: Flexibility exercises aim to improve the range of motion and mobility of the joints and muscles. These exercises can include activities such as yoga, Pilates, and tai chi. Flexibility exercises have been shown to improve posture, balance, and body awareness, as well as reduce the risk of injury and improve overall physical and mental well-being[5].

4. **Balance and Stability Exercise**: Balance and stability exercises focus on improving the body's

ability to maintain balance and stability, which can be achieved through activities such as yoga, Pilates, and tai chi. These exercises have been shown to improve proprioception, coordination, and overall balance, as well as reduce the risk of falls and injuries, and improve overall physical and mental well-being.

- Exercise and Neuroplasticity

Exercise and neuroplasticity are interconnected concepts that play a significant role in the mind-gut immune connection. Neuroplasticity refers to the brain's ability to form new connections, adapt, and reorganize itself throughout life. Exercise has been shown to have a positive impact on neuroplasticity, leading to improvements in cognitive function, learning, and memory.

Physical exercise has been found to enhance neuroplasticity and cognitive function in several ways:

1. **Increased Neurotrophic Factors**: Exercise has been shown to increase the expression of brain-derived neurotrophic factor (BDNF), a protein that promotes the growth and maintenance of nerve cells. BDNF plays a crucial role in the development of new neurons and the strengthening of existing ones, and is essential for learning and memory.

2. **Neuroprotection**: Exercise has been found to promote neuroprotection, which is the brain's ability to resist damage and recover from injuries. This protection is thought to be due to the unique capability of the skeletal muscle to increase activation to the cellular signaling pathways connected to crosstalk between muscle and brain.

3. **Improved Learning and Memory**: Exercise has been shown to improve learning and memory by promoting the formation of new memories and enhancing the retrieval of existing ones. This improvement in cognitive function is thought to be due to the increased production of BDNF and other neurotrophic factors.

4. **Reduced Inflammation**: Exercise has been found to reduce inflammation in the brain, which is known to contribute to cognitive decline and neurodegenerative diseases such as Alzheimer's and Parkinson's. Reducing inflammation can help preserve cognitive function and promote overall brain health.

5. **Regulation of Microglia**: Exercise has been shown to affect the structure and function of microglia, the major immune cells in the central nervous system. Exercise has been reported to decrease the aging-induced activation and proliferation of microglia in the hippocampus, which is a region of the brain involved in learning and memory.

- Exercise Prescription

Exercise prescription refers to the development of individualized plans for physical activity that aim to improve health, prevent disease, and enhance overall well-being. In the context of the mind-gut immune connection, exercise prescription can play a crucial role in promoting overall health and well-being by influencing the gut microbiota and immune system.

Research has shown that engaging in exercise can lead to a specific microbial profile in the gut that is associated with improved health outcomes. Exercise has been found to alter the gut microbiota in humans with overweight and obesity, leading to a healthier gut environment. Additionally, home-based exercise training has been shown to influence gut bacterial levels in individuals with multiple sclerosis, suggesting that even modest-intensity exercise can have a positive impact on gut health.

Endurance exercise has also been found to have effects on gut microbiota, including the correction of electrolyte imbalances and modulation of the immune response during intense physical activity. These effects can contribute to a more balanced and healthy gut environment, which in turn can support the immune system and overall health.

Conclusion

This examination of the mind-gut-immune relationship has been a fascinating exploration of the delicate interplay of three essential systems that define our total health and well-being. We've explored neuroscience, gastroenterology, immunology, and psychoneuroimmunology, uncovering a tapestry of links that highlight the tremendous influence our mental moods, gut health, and immune function have on one another.

Reflecting on our full understanding, it is clear that maintaining a healthy balance among the mind, stomach, and immune system is critical for overall health. With its bidirectional communication, the mind-gut axis exposes the significant effect of thoughts and emotions on digestive processes, as well as how the state of the gut may shape mental well-being. As a vigilant watchdog, the immune system stands at the crossroads, responding to signals from both the mind and the gut, underlining the interconnection of both systems.

The investigation of the current research environment has revealed the field's dynamic character. From neuroscientific breakthroughs tracing neuronal networks between the brain and the stomach to game-changing findings in gut microbiota and immunology, the scientific community is constantly revealing new levels of understanding. As the study of the mind-body link, psychoneuroimmunology has produced important insights into the influence of stress, emotions, and neurological pathways on immunological responses, setting the groundwork for creative approaches to holistic health.

Discussions on tailored wellness programs, nutrient-rich meals, and lifestyle choices that support a robust mind-gut-immune axis have been a cornerstone of this journey. Mindfulness, stress reduction, and the incorporation of good bacteria via probiotics are not just theoretical notions; they are concrete steps toward improving the interrelated health of these important systems.

The changing panorama of mind-gut-immune research holds promise for tailored interventions and innovative therapies in the future. Recognizing the importance of resilience and the role of each individual in actively designing their health journey, we emphasize the value of individual heterogeneity in responses.

In summary, this comprehensive book aims to provide readers with the knowledge and skills they need to make educated decisions regarding their food, lifestyle, and mental health. It emphasizes the tremendous influence of these decisions on the mind, stomach, and immune system, ultimately leading people along a road of holistic health and well-being. Once recognized and cultivated, the mind-gut-immune link becomes a powerful ally in the quest of a balanced and fulfilling existence.